Carpal Tunnel

How To Treat Carpal Tunnel Syndrome
How To Prevent
Carpal Tunnel Syndrome

By Ace McCloud
Copyright © 2013

Disclaimer

The information provided in this book is designed to provide helpful information on the subjects discussed. This book is not meant to be used, nor should it be used, to diagnose or treat any medical condition. For diagnosis or treatment of any medical problem, consult your own physician. The publisher and author are not responsible for any specific health or allergy needs that may require medical supervision and are not liable for any damages or negative consequences from any treatment, action, application or preparation, to any person reading or following the information in this book. Any references included are provided for informational purposes only. Readers should be aware that any websites or links listed in this book may change.

Table of Contents

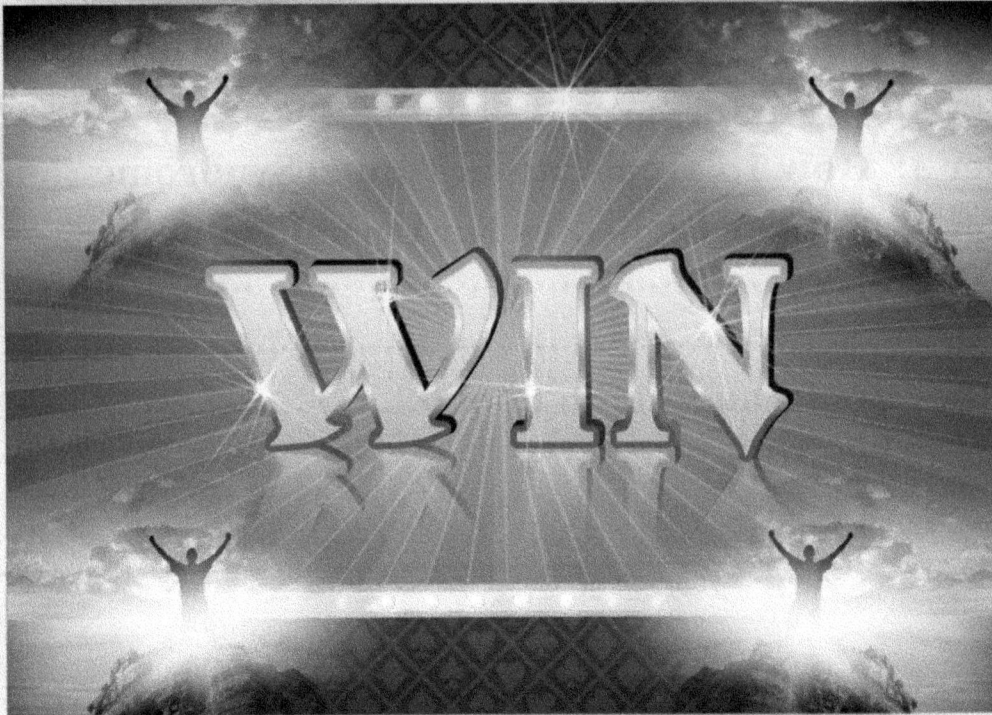

DEDICATED TO THOSE WHO ARE PLAYING THE GAME OF LIFE TO

WIN

KEEP ON PUSHING AND NEVER GIVE UP!

Ace McCloud

Be sure to check out my website for all my Books and Audio books.

www.AcesEbooks.com

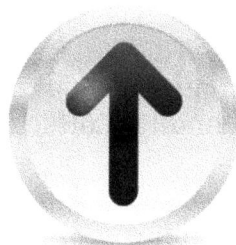

Introduction

I want to thank you and congratulate you for buying the book, "Carpal Tunnel Syndrome Solution: Diagnosing Carpal Tunnel Syndrome, How To Prevent Carpal Tunnel Syndrome, and How To Treat Carpal Tunnel Syndrome."

This book contains proven steps and strategies on how to diagnose, prevent, and treat carpal tunnel syndrome, a condition afflicting many individuals around the world.

Along with an overview of carpal tunnel syndrome, which includes factors believed to cause it and how to diagnose it correctly, this book will clearly outline the best prevention practices, along with doctor-prescribed and alternative treatments. Anyone looking to better understand carpal tunnel syndrome will benefit immensely from reading this book.

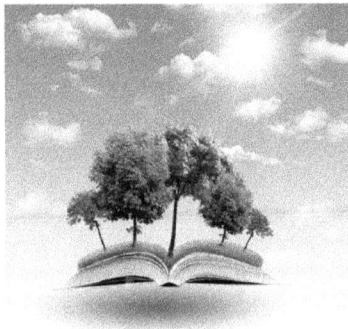

Chapter 1: Overview of Carpal Tunnel Syndrome

Carpal Tunnel Syndrome, also known as CTS, is a condition that is brought about by the pinching of the nerve in the wrist. The median nerve, as this nerve is called, runs from the brain and spinal cord all the way to the tips of the fingers, and is what allows the brain to communicate with the hands.

The condition earned the name because of the tunnel-like structure of the median nerve as it passes through in the wrist area: a tight ligament at the top, and the wrist bones at the bottom, both of which are extremely inflexible structures. Because of this, when there is a buildup of pressure in the carpal tunnel area, the nerve, pushing up against rigid material on all sides, has nowhere to go. It gets squished, causing it to function improperly.

Allowing this condition to persist can lead to several short term and long term consequences for you. Along with pain, tingling, and feelings of numbness, primarily in the fingers and hands area, leaving your carpal tunnel syndrome untreated can cause permanent medial nerve damage.

Over time, you may experience a decrease in grip strength, as the muscles of the hand begin to atrophy. The severity of your pain and cramping will also increase, as the nerve begins to deteriorate due to the tremendous swelling around it. Your nerve impulses may slow down, you may lose feeling in your fingers, and lose coordination and strength at the bottom of your thumb area. Eventually, untreated CTS can result in permanent muscle tissue deterioration, and ultimately, complete loss of all hand functions. If part of the reason for your carpal tunnel systems is from being online all the time or excessive playing of video games, you should definitely check out my book on Internet and Gaming Addiction.

While the link between repetitive movements and carpal tunnel syndrome is still not fully verified, employees who work in places that require repetitive tasks to be performed with their hands tend to experience the longest absences from their jobs and have a lower production rate due to the symptoms described above.

Chapter 2: How To Diagnose Carpal Tunnel Syndrome

While there are a host of symptoms that you can experience due to CTS, the telltale signs all revolve around pain, tingling, and numbness in the hand and fingers area. The most common symptoms include pain in the hand and wrist area, a feeling of weakness in certain hand muscles, and unusual tingling and numbing sensations in particular areas of the hand. Additionally, people suffering from CTS often comment that shaking their hand forcefully tends to relieve their symptoms temporarily.

While the areas affected from pain tend to be in the hand and wrist, the feelings of hurt may spread to the lower and even the upper arm. Pain is also generally reported as being more acute at night, possibly because some people turn over during their sleep and end up with their hand underneath them, with the full weight of their body on top of it.

To be certain that you have CTS and not just temporary feelings of pain, tingling, and numbness, there are some tests that either you or medical professionals can administer for a more complete diagnosis.

The first such exam is called Tinel's Test. To perform Tinel's Test, the median nerve is tapped along it's path through the wrist. A worsening of the tingling sensation in the fingers during this test would indicate a possibly positive result for carpal tunnel syndrome.

The second such exam is called Phalen's Test. To perform this test, push the back of your hands tightly together for one full minute. Doing so will compress the carpal tunnel area, and if the symptoms you've experienced thus far get worse, the test has indicated a positive result.

A third such exam, called Durkan's Test, consists of applying firm pressure for up to thirty seconds to the palm area directly over the nerve. As with the previous two tests, a continuation or heightening of symptoms would mean the test has returned a positive result as well.

A more technical examination would involve sending electric impulses along the median nerve, and then looking for irregularities in nerve impulse conduction with a machine called an EMG. Given that the EMG exam is more involved, since it requires a visit to a medical professional, it does not typically need to be administered. However, if the symptoms you are experiencing are extremely severe or painful, an EMG exam may be necessary.

The causes of the compression of the carpal tunnel area, and thus carpal tunnel syndrome, continue to create controversy throughout the medical community, as a consensus has yet to be reached. Arthritis, diabetes, prediabetes (imperfect glucose tolerance) hypothyroidism, pregnancy, obesity, oral contraceptives, and trauma all are thought to bring on the onset of CTS. Also, repetitive movements of the fingers from typing, playing video games, or any other repetitive task using the hands and fingers over long periods of time is strongly linked to carpal tunnel syndrome. Genetics can also play a part in developing CTS.

Some researchers believe that the condition can be caused by intrinsic and extrinsic factors exerting pressure from both inside and outside of the tunnel. Benign tumors in the wrist area, for example, are one such factor that could aid the condition in developing.

Given the exponential increase in computer usage over the last couple of decades, the mouse and keyboard have become targets of blame for patients who suffer from CTS. Many believe that the repeated finger and wrist movements required for typing and mouse clicking can compress the tunnel area, pinching the median nerve. Correspondingly, other activities that involve repetitive finger and wrist movements, such as tennis, weightlifting, video games, and industrial shop work have been linked to carpal tunnel syndrome.

Chapter 3: How To Prevent Carpal Tunnel Syndrome

Regardless of whether the medical community will soon reach an agreement as to the causes of carpal tunnel syndrome, anyone who spends a large amount of time in front of a computer should develop good work habits, such as having good posture and putting their monitor at eye level, which can help prevent other ailments such as lower back pain and eye strain.

Visit your local office supply store, computer store, or simply browse online to find an ergonomically designed keyboard, mouse, wrist pads, and chair that will allow you to preserve excellent posture and reduce strain on your hands while working at your computer.

In order to help-prevent injuries, try to do a five minute hand warm-up before you start working, in the same way runners stretch before commencing a run. To help prevent carpal tunnel syndrome, there are a number of simple exercises that can be done.

Hand Exercises

Stand up, with your arms extended fully out in front of you, with the back of your hand facing you. Extend and stretch your wrists and fingers, and hold for five seconds.
Next, straighten both of your wrists and relax your fingers, letting them hang limply towards the ground.
Then, with both hands, make a tight fist. Continuing to keep your arms fully extended out, point your fists down towards the ground and hold for another five seconds.
Unclench your fists, straighten both wrists, and allow your fingers to hang loosely down again.
Repeat the movements ten times, and when you are done, allow your arms to hang loosely at your side, shaking them slightly for a couple of seconds each.

Another great exercise you can try involves pushing on the top of your fingers. While standing or sitting, extend one arm fully out in front of you, with your palm facing forward. With your other hand, pull the tops of your fingers back towards yourself in a slow, tugging motion. You should feel a stretch in the underside of your wrist. Try to do at least fifteen reps on each hand at least six times per day.

A third exercise requires you to extend one arm out to the side (slightly less than parallel with the ground), with your palm facing up. Gently angle your fingers down towards the floor. As you do this, you should feel a tightening of your forearm muscles. Lastly, tilt your head away from your extended arm, trying to touch your ear to your shoulder. Hold for thirty seconds, and repeat three times for each arm. As you become more limber, you can push your hand up against the wall for a greater stretch.

This last exercise can help alleviate pain or tingling sensations in the shoulder area due to CTS. Drape a towel over whichever shoulder is causing you problems, grabbing it in front of you at belly button level with one hand, and also behind you with the other hand. Gently pull down with each hand, stretching the towel out, and slowly tilt your head away from the towel. Hold for thirty seconds, and repeat three times with each shoulder (if needed).

Setting Up Your Work Area

Posture

To ensure good posture, computer users should always sit up tall, pushing the hips as far back as they can go. Seat height should be adjusted so that the feet sit flatly on the ground, with the knee height equal to (or slightly lower than) the hips. If the chair can be reclined, adjust it to make an angle of between 100 and 110 degrees. To ensure that both the upper and lower back are supported, make use of inflatable cushions or small pillows, and position the armrests (if present) so that the shoulders are in a relaxed position. If the armrests prove too uncomfortable, simply remove them from the chair.

Keyboard Placement

To achieve proper keyboard placement, sit as close to it as possible, ensuring that the keyboard is centered with your chest. Also keep in mind that the shoulders need to be relaxed, adjust the keyboard height so that your elbows end up slightly open, and your wrists and hands are straight. You may have to tilt your keyboard away from you if you sit in a forward or upright position. Conversely, if you sit in a slightly reclined position, then your keyboard should be tilted slightly forward so as to allow the wrists to remain straight. Such positioning can be achieved either by using the keyboard tray mechanism, or by using the keyboard feet found underneath it. You can also buy keyboard trays that will attach to your desk allowing for proper placement of the mouse and keyboard. These keyboard trays are highly recommended.

Wrist Rests

Wrist rests are also a worthwhile purchase, as they will assist in padding hard desk surfaces and maintaining good posture. Keep in mind, however, that typing should not be done while resting on the wrist rests, as they should only be used for resting between keystrokes. Also, try to position your mouse as near to the keyboard as possible.

Computer Gloves

I used to wear the big carpal tunnel gloves that went halfway up your forearm and had the metal brace on the underneath. I found that over time, the metal brace would dig into my hand and cause bruising and pain. I just recently bought some computer gloves and love them! I have put my old clunky old carpal tunnel gloves in the storage bin and replaced them with some gloves that are really making a difference. They are called Imak computer gloves. They fit the hand very comfortably, are reversible, washable, and have a very cool cushion made of beads that helps protect the wrist area. I would highly recommend these gloves if you are on the computer over two hours a day.

Foot Pedals

Foot pedals are also a wise investment. These are electronic foot pedals that sit on the ground and that can be programmed to replicate any keyboard or mouse command. I personally got my foot pedals online and have programmed them to replicate mouse clicks. The ones I got have two pedals. I have programmed the left pedal to replicate a left mouse click and the right pedal to replicate a right mouse click. This can save you a ton of unnecessary hand movements throughout a normal workday and it is actually sort of fun clicking with your feet.

Voice Recognition Software

Another electronic device that can save your hands a ton of aggravation is voice recognition software. This type of software allows you to talk into a microphone and it will type whatever you say onto the screen. This can save your hands from a lot of unnecessary movements and pain over the long-term. I like to use the newest version of Dragon NaturallySpeaking voice recognition software. I found that it works incredibly well. I use it on e-mails, when I'm writing, and for most anything else that requires typing on a computer. This could be one your best investments for saving your hands from untold amounts of typing and aggravation.

Gaming Keyboard

A gaming keyboard can also save your hands a lot of wear and tear. If you do play video games on the computer, a gaming keyboard can be programmed to do a variety of keystrokes or mouse commands that will really save your hands from a lot of damage. Even if you don't play video games on the computer, you can program a gaming keyboard for all the different user names and passwords that you use. I have two keyboards plugged in at the same time. The first is an ergonomic keyboard that is easy on the hands and is what I use primarily. The second is a gaming keyboard that has all of my most common user names and passwords programmed into it so that with just the press of one button I can access my favorite programs and places on the internet. Logitech makes great gaming keyboards.

Monitor Position

Positioning the monitor properly can also help with good computer usage posture. In order to keep your neck in a relaxed position, the monitor should be centered directly in front of your eyes, about an arm's length away, with the top of the monitor two to three inches above eye level. Lower the monitor to a comfortable reading level if you wear bifocals. And if needed, open or close curtains or blinds to minimize glare.

Document Positioning

If you are reading off of a document, position it so that it sits directly in front of you. If there is sufficient space, put the document on a holder. Additionally, place your telephone within arm's reach from your sitting position to avoid over extending. Also, utilizing headsets or the speaker feature on a phone allows you to stay in the correct posture to eliminate unnecessary strain on your neck and body.

Planned Breaks

To release pent up muscle tension that can develop after prolonged computer usage, take small breaks frequently throughout the day (ideally every thirty minutes). There is a long list of scientific research showing that sitting for long periods of time, whether driving, typing, or just being on the computer in general, can be very damaging to your health. During these break periods, walk around or consider doing some light stretches. It is also a great time to do some of the hand exercises mentioned earlier. As a general rule, avoid ordering out for lunch so that you can give yourself a chance to get away from your desk. And so as to not wear out your eyes, refocus them periodically, focusing on something far off in the distance instead of at the up-close monitor.

Doing the simple exercises mentioned earlier in this chapter, while using some of the helpful tips, devices, and posture techniques mentioned above, may be enough to prevent you from experiencing the pain and discomfort associated with CTS, and if you already have it, they should help relieve your symptoms dramatically.

Chapter 4: How To Treat Carpal Tunnel Syndrome

As with any condition, moderate and conservative treatments should be tried first before turning to invasive surgical procedures. To help decrease the inflammation associated with carpal tunnel (and also the symptoms associated with it), consider taking anti-inflammatory medications, also known as NSAID's, such as Advil.

You can also wear a wrist brace or computer gloves to support the wrist area. In the neutral position (wrist level), the carpal tunnel will be at its widest diameter, exerting the least amount of pressure on the median nerve. Be sure to wear the brace or gloves while doing repetitive hand and finger activities, and possibly at night as well while sleeping if the symptoms are severe enough.

If symptoms persist, ask your physician about cortisone injections to the affected area. Cortisone injections tend to be effective about eighty percent of the time. Unfortunately, the relief cortisone injections provide tends to be only temporary, as symptoms usually return within a year's time. In addition, any steroid treatment should be used sparingly, as harmful side effects can develop from prolonged use.

If the pain and discomfort continue to worsen, surgery may be required to alleviate the inflammation. The most common surgical procedure is known as the carpal tunnel release. By making a small incision in the sheath surrounding the carpal tunnel, pressure is released, thereby easing the tension on the median nerve. This procedure tends to be done using an "open" technique, where the performing surgeon makes a small incision (typically around four centimeters) down the middle of the palm, and proceeds to peel away the hand tissue until the carpal tunnel is accessible. The procedure is very short, taking only about fifteen minutes, and can be done with local, regional, or general anesthesia.

With the advent of microscopic cameras, a carpal tunnel release can now be performed without having to open up the palm area. During an endoscopic carpal tunnel release, a small incision (typically one centimeter) is made in the wrist area. The camera is then inserted into the carpal tunnel, with a small knife attached. Being able to view the area on a screen, the performing surgeon uses the small knife to ease the tension around the carpal tunnel.

While both procedures are effective in decreasing swelling, many surgeons report complications from the invasive carpal tunnel release. Among the problems reported are the accidental cutting of a nerve, and a longer healing time. Roughly five to eight percent of all surgeries will result in injury to the nerve, which may create a permanent area of numbness towards the base of the thumb. In about one to two percent of cases, patients report feelings of prolonged pain at the point of incision.

Chapter 5: Natural Remedies For Carpal Tunnel Syndrome

While conventional medicines and procedures are rather effective for treating carpal tunnel syndrome, the potential side effects may make you consider seeking alternative treatment options.

Proper nutrition is a simple and easy way to treat the carpal tunnel symptoms. To help reduce inflammation, consume Vitamin B6 and Lipoic Acid. A deficiency of Vitamin B6 could be a cause of CTS, so be sure to get tested for that deficiency. Foods like potatoes, sweet potatoes, brown rice, chickpeas, pork, avocados, chicken, beef, turkey, barley, mangoes, bananas, and sunflower seeds are foods you may want to consider adding to your diet for additional B6 nutrients. However, since most foods contain only a small amount of B6, you may not notice a change in your symptoms for weeks or even months. Taking vitamin supplements, then, is considered the most effective and quickest way to raise your Vitamin B6 level. Be sure to always seek the advice of a qualified physician to help monitor your vitamin intake, since too much B6 can lead to serious side effects, such as neurological problems.

Other foods that should be consumed in your diet are whole grains, nuts, seeds, and vegetables. Also, foods such as pineapples, wild fish fat, red palm oil, cruciferous vegetables (such as broccoli and red cabbage), berries, and turmeric are known to be anti-inflammatory and will therefore help reduce swelling.

As far as foods to avoid, the general rule of thumb applies. Fried foods, and those high in saturated fat are a poor diet choice, as are those that contain yellow (hydrazine) dyes. Furthermore, having a large intake of alcohol, caffeine, and tobacco is believed to be associated with the onset of CTS.

If you seek an herbal remedy, consider taking wild yam, black pepper, cayenne, chives, basil, rosemary, St. John's Wort, Turmeric, cramp bark, willow bark, and Bromelain in any form. All are believed to help ease the pain and minimize the swelling due to carpal tunnel syndrome.

If you do not have a serious aversion to needles, acupuncture is a viable alternative treatment option for carpal tunnel. Once blocked pathways can be opened with tiny needles, and normal nerve function can be returned to the wrist area. In addition to the hands area, acupuncturists can treat the meridians (body lines that contain hundreds of acupuncture points) of the liver, gallbladder, and kidney.

Instead of acupuncture, which involves needles, you may prefer acupressure, which is simply applying pressure to certain points on the body that are in need of stimulation. Visiting a chiropractor may also prove to be a good option.

Massage for CTS

Massage therapy is also an excellent option. There are experts who know how to massage you to relieve painful symptoms. Even if they are not an expert at treating CTS, just making sure they spend 15 minutes or more working specifically on your hands, fingers, wrists, forearms, and arms will be a big help. This is one of the most effective methods for treatment if you can afford it, and there are tons of healing benefits associated with massage therapy.

A good massage technique that you can do yourself involves applying pressure directly to the wrist area. Bend your arm in front of you at ninety degrees, with your palm facing up. Take your other hand, and place your thumb on top of the wrist, and your pointer finger (or any other finger) below the wrist. Slowly rub into the wrist with your thumb using long circular movements.

Next, once you feel the muscles start to loosen, begin to move your fingers up the forearm towards the elbow. Try rubbing in a side-to-side motion across the forearm in addition to moving in a circular pattern.

Also, try keeping your fingers locked and move them up the forearm, from the wrist to the elbow, as if you were smoothing out a wrinkle in a bed sheet by pushing it towards the edge.

If your condition requires it, move all the way up the arm, passing over the bicep area and onto the shoulder. Once at the shoulder, push directly into it (near the armpit area) to help ease the stress caused by carpal tunnel syndrome.

For More information on Massage Therapy, Trigger Point Therapy and Acupressure that you can do on your own, be sure to check out my book: Massage Therapy, Trigger Point Therapy, and Acupressure.

Other Therapies

The idea behind hydrotherapy is that by applying hot and cold water compresses, the contrast can provide some relief for those who suffer from CTS. Fully submerge your wrists in hot water for three minutes, followed by one minute in cold water. Repeat three times. Throughout the day, try and perform the whole process at least two or three times. A great re-usable hot/cold pack is: Nexcare Reusable Hot/Cold Pack.

Hypnotherapy is another alternative treatment. Under hypnosis, you may be able to access the body's inner healing mechanisms, thereby eradicating the aches and pains associated with CTS. I highly recommend Hypnosis Downloads for this. A good download is called: Pain Relief.

Considered an effective treatment for many physical maladies, yoga may prove highly effective for treating carpal tunnel syndrome. The choreographed poses and deep, slow breathing of yoga are perfect for relaxing and dealing with chronic pain, while at the same time strengthening and stretching muscles and joints to ease tension.

Cool, damp weather is believed to amplify CTS symptoms. If moving to a warmer climate, or even raising the thermostat at home or at work, is not an option, consider wearing fingerless gloves so that you can still have full functionality of your hands while keeping them and your wrists warm.

Lastly, be aware of the amount of force you use for tasks such as typing. Many people use a lot more force than is required when pressing the keys. Also, when opening things such as jars, try not to use your thumb and forefinger. Instead, utilize your entire hand, which will take some of the pressure off of the wrist area. Lastly, try to use your non-dominant hand more often, such as with the mouse. This will give your dominant hand a break, and make developing CTS symptoms less likely.

My Personal Strategies

Right before I know I will be using my hands a lot, I will take a large pot and fill it with fairly hot water. Not so hot that it burns, but pretty hot. I will then soak my hands in it for five minutes. Feel free to add Epsom salts to the hot water, but it is not required. The next thing I will do is stretch out my hands and fingers using the exercises described earlier in the book. I also like to do about thirty wrist curls with a light weight dumbbell, and then use a grip ball to really get my hands strong and loose.

I will then apply some Penetrex cream to my hands. I can honestly say that Penetrex is nothing short of miraculous. I can't recommend it enough. Instead of other creams that relieve pain, this cream actually works by healing your hands! Nothing I have ever tried or done works as good as this cream! After the hot water soak, hand stretches, and applying the Penetrex, I put on my Imak computer gloves, and get to work. I am also careful to take breaks every twenty to thirty minutes, and I make sure that I am stretching out my hands during those breaks.

I used to ice my hands throughout the day, but I found this did not work very well if there was more work that I needed to do with my hands. I found it was better for me to use heat and stretching when using my hands a lot, and then to ice my hands and forearms in a large bucket of ice water at night or when I wouldn't be using my hands for several hours.

Conclusion

I hope this book was able to help you become much more knowledgeable in dealing with and curing your carpal tunnel syndrome.

By utilizing all the information and techniques outlined in this book it should make it much less likely that you will develop carpal tunnel syndrome, and if you have it already, it should help you greatly reduce its negative effects. Be sure to do the stretching exercises every day, especially before you are about to do a lot of work with your hands, and remember to use everything at your disposal to make the work load on your hands easier! I especially love the voice recognition software and using the foot pedals to do mouse clicking. If you work at it, your pain should be a thing of the past and you will be able to function at much higher levels without being held back by your carpal tunnel syndrome.

Finally, if you discovered at least one thing that has helped you or that you think would be beneficial to someone else, be sure to take a few seconds to easily post a quick positive review. As an author, your positive feedback is desperately needed. Your highly valuable five star reviews are like a river of golden joy flowing through a sunny forest of mighty trees and beautiful flowers! *To do your good deed in making the world a better place by helping others with your valuable insight, just leave a nice review.*

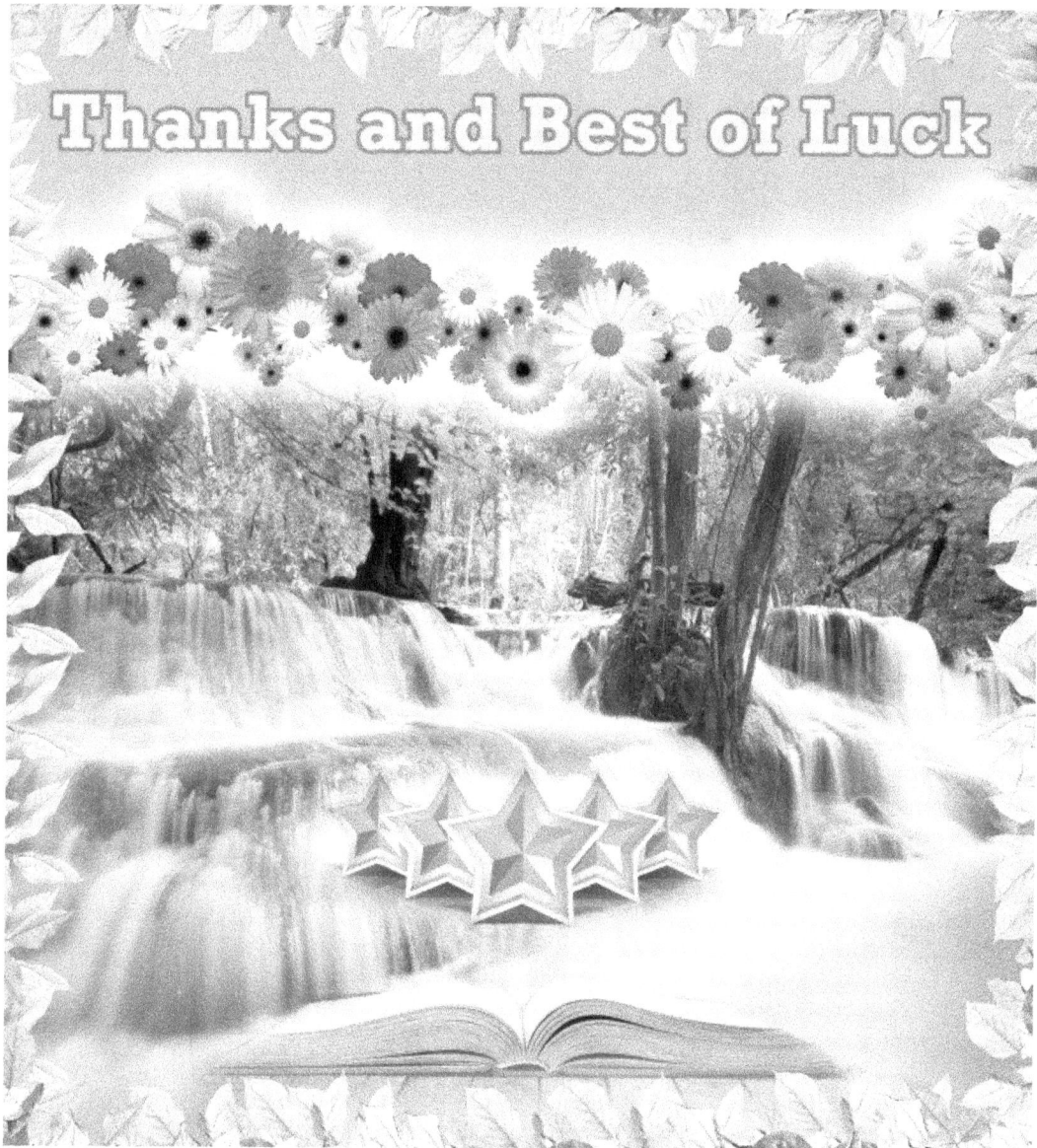

Thanks and Best of Luck

My Other Books and Audio Books

Health Books

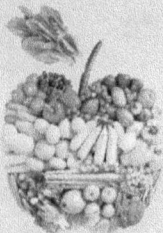

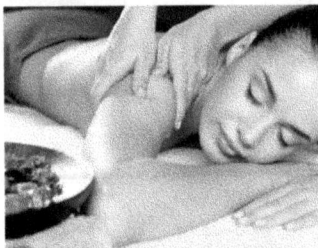

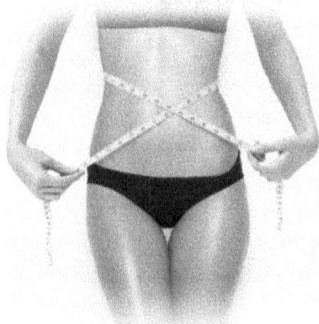

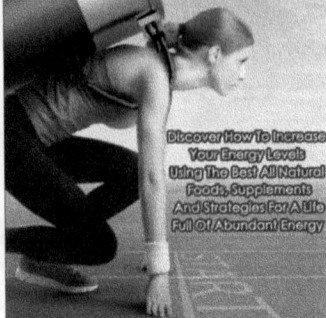

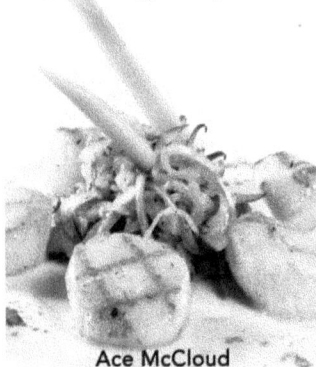

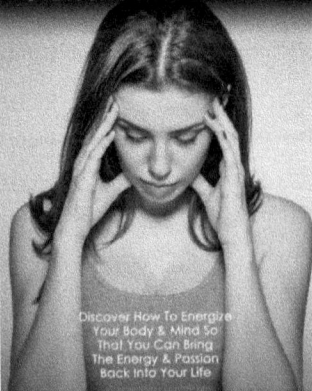

Peak Performance Books

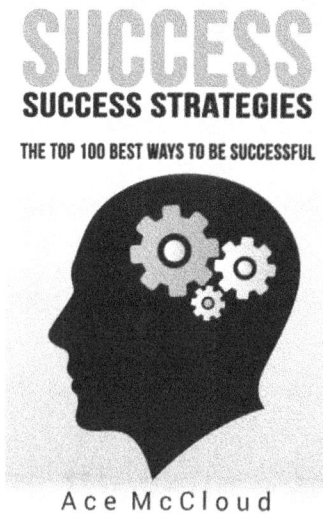

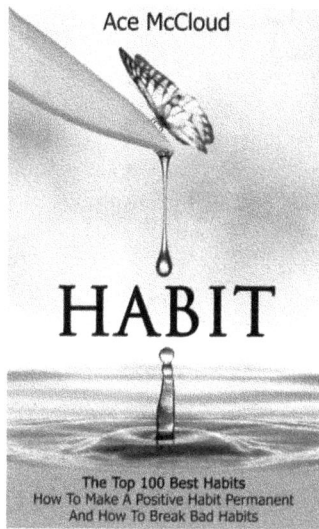

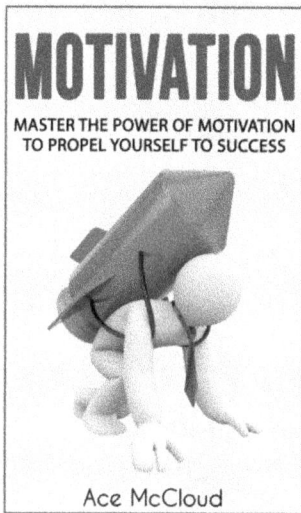

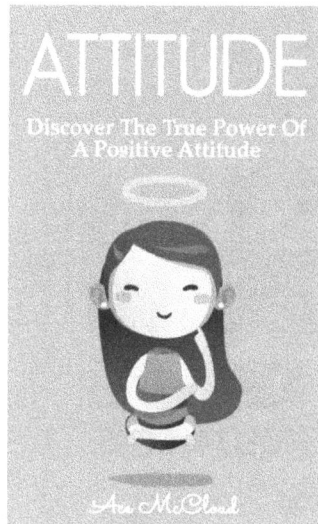

SUCCESS
SUCCESS STRATEGIES
THE TOP 100 BEST WAYS TO BE SUCCESSFUL

Ace McCloud

Ace McCloud

HABIT

The Top 100 Best Habits
How To Make A Positive Habit Permanent
And How To Break Bad Habits

MOTIVATION
MASTER THE POWER OF MOTIVATION TO PROPEL YOURSELF TO SUCCESS

Ace McCloud

ATTITUDE
Discover The True Power Of A Positive Attitude

Ace McCloud

SELF DISCIPLINE

Unleash The Power Of Self Discipline, Influence And Willpower In Your Life To Achieve Anything

Ace McCloud

Competitive Strategies

WINNING STRATEGIES

The Top 100 Best Strategies For Peak Performance During Competitions

Ace McCloud

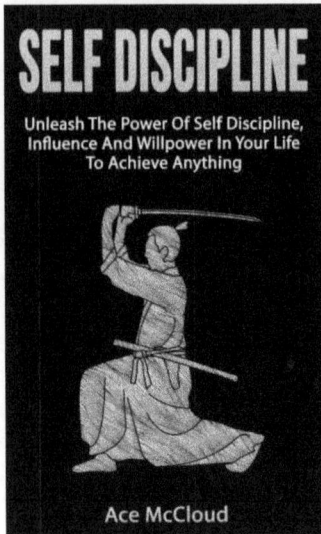

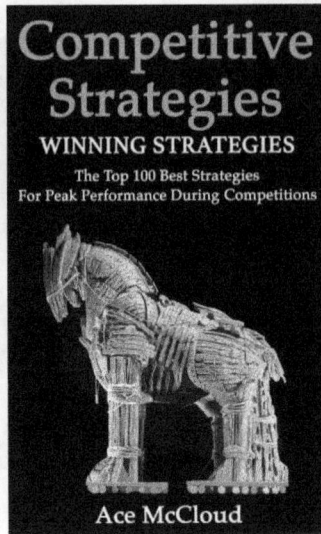

Be sure to check out my audio books as well!

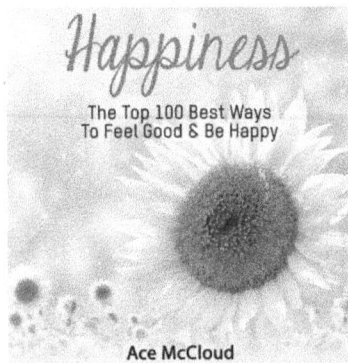

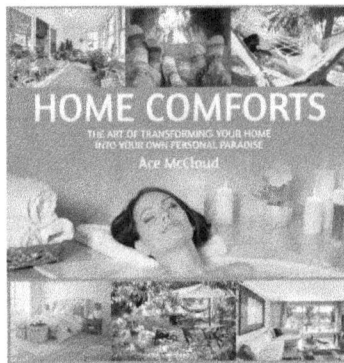

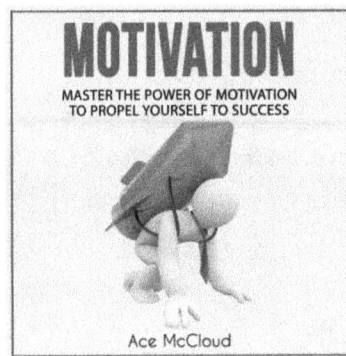

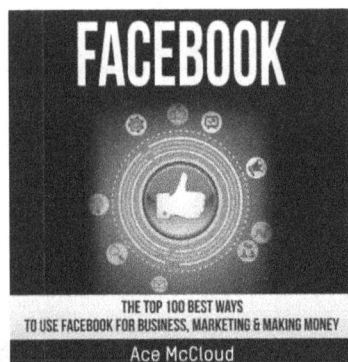

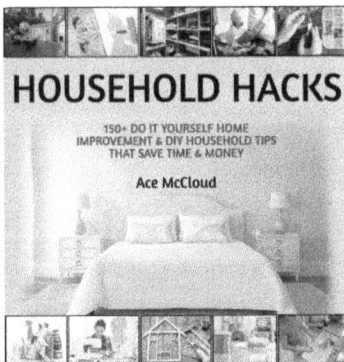

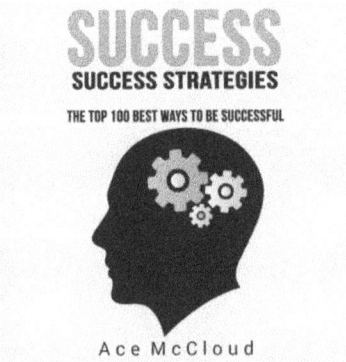

Happiness

The Top 100 Best Ways To Feel Good & Be Happy

Ace McCloud

HOME COMFORTS

THE ART OF TRANSFORMING YOUR HOME INTO YOUR OWN PERSONAL PARADISE

Ace McCloud

MOTIVATION

MASTER THE POWER OF MOTIVATION TO PROPEL YOURSELF TO SUCCESS

Ace McCloud

FACEBOOK

THE TOP 100 BEST WAYS TO USE FACEBOOK FOR BUSINESS, MARKETING & MAKING MONEY

Ace McCloud

HOUSEHOLD HACKS

150+ DO IT YOURSELF HOME IMPROVEMENT & DIY HOUSEHOLD TIPS THAT SAVE TIME & MONEY

Ace McCloud

SUCCESS

SUCCESS STRATEGIES

THE TOP 100 BEST WAYS TO BE SUCCESSFUL

Ace McCloud

Check out my website at: www.AcesEbooks.com for a complete list of all of my books and high quality audio books. I enjoy bringing you the best knowledge in the world and wish you the best in using this information to make your journey through life better and more enjoyable! **Best of luck to you!**